The Wheelc

"In It to Win It"

By Sonja P. Davis

ROYSTON
Publishing

BK Royston Publishing
P. O. Box 4321
Jeffersonville, IN 47131
502-802-5385
http://www.bkroystonpublishing.com
bkroystonpublishing@gmail.com

Cover Design: Keshia Webb and Kamaal Designs
Photo Credit: Raynetta Curd (Ray Ray)

ISBN-10:1-946111-35-X
ISBN-13:978-1-946111-35-7

Printed in the United States of America

Dedication

To anyone who's tired and ready to give up, **don't!**

To anyone who thinks they can't make it, **you can**!

To anyone who's broken, can't pray and feels all alone. **You are never alone. Someone somewhere has you on their mind and they're praying for you.**

To anyone who needs understanding. You find yourself searching here, there and everywhere for answers; just trying to find a reason why certain things happen. **Take out your Bible. Read it. You'll find your answer**.

To anyone who asks these questions: Why me? What am I supposed to do? Why this? Why now? When is it going to end? **Just Pray! Be still and know He is God. He will work it out.**

To anyone, anywhere going through anything, **no matter what it is.**

I know that when I pray, God hears me and He answers my prayers. And I'm truly grateful, because something marvelous happens for the person I'm praying for and something amazing happens for me as well.

This book is my offering to you.

Stay focused; Keep the Faith, and Keep Going

Acknowledgments

Editor and Publisher: BK Royston Publishing. Julia, it was your organization that read my manuscript and said, "My story was powerful and needed to be heard." Your service to others will help meet the needs of God's people and it will create an appreciation of gratefulness to God. Thank you and I pray God blesses you and your organization for blessing me.

Tonie Carol Courtney. You are my Best Friend and sister for 40 years. Sis, you've always stood by myside. Whether I'm right or wrong, you let me know either way. That means more to me than anything, keeping it real; gracefully. You speak from your heart and that's the place where God dwells. Sis, you believe in goodness, kindness and honesty. That my dear friend, I will always treasure. The bond we share as sisters is a blessing from God. I love you and thank God for you.

Wendy Goodwin. You are my Angel and sister for 30 years. Sis, we've connected spiritually at work and kept it real from the very first day we met; you've never changed. Recently, your encouraging words touched me more than ever. You said, "Sis, I wish I could bear some of what you're going through, but the blessings that are going to come are not for me; they are for you." You told me to hold on with faith and to keep my eyes on our Gracious and Merciful Savior Jesus Christ! You are my Dearest friend and I thank God for you and cherish you.

Sheila Bivens aka Sheila B. You are my Beloved and loyal friend for over 25 years. Girlfriend, there's nobody like you. It was you while I was in Frazier Rehab that gathered a few of our close friends together from Lace Social Club (Tonya Calvert, Tyra Cole and Octavia Johnson) from back in the day, to surprise me. It felt so good reconnecting and fellowshipping, and on top of that having a Topshelf Caterer; Maurice J. Eddie owner of Table 4 2 Catering Service LLC and Decorations. More importantly, I was blessed to find out that my husband and daughter was part of making this surprise possible. Also, Sherise Leslie and Connie Page were involved in this surprise as well. Words cannot express the love I felt in that conference room. Only God can reward you in this life time for all the love you have shown and the lives you touched. I got you Sheila B. Just keep being you. It doesn't go unnoticed. I love you and thank God for you.

Debra Rowe Ross. My sister soldier and dependable girlfriend for over 25 years. First, of all thank you for serving in the military. Sis, you came into my life with boldness, faith and confidence; especially, when it came to the Word of God. You are my prayer warrior. You inspire me and keep me encouraged, which is the fuel that I need to keep on going. Thank you, girlfriend, for blessing me and keeping it real; no matter what. I love you and thank God for you.

Angie Bush Ross. My diamond and pearl red hat diva sister, traveling partner, and fabulous girlfriend. Sis, we've been traveling together for over 20 years. The bond we share on the road is never the same when I travel with anyone else. We were 2 broke sisters enjoying life as if we had at all. The fun we share looking stunning and glamorous is awesome, especially, when we go to a HBCU Homecoming at Kentucky State University. The love, the fellowship, the distinction, and the ultimate turn-up is like being at an HBCU family reunion. Sis, thank you for caring for me and embracing with love. Girlfriend, the bond we share and the friends I met through you will always be in my heart forever. I love you and thank God for you.

Patricia Daniels. My motivator. Sis, you are the one who motivated me to go back to school. And because of you I attended colleges that offered a Christ-centered learning environment designed for working adults. I earned 3 Degrees. An MBA from Ottawa University, including, an ASB & BSM (magna cum laude) from Indiana Wesleyan University. Thank you for motivating me for over 25 years and being available for me when I needed you. I love you and thank God for you.

Paula Thornton. My reliable girlfriend. Sis, I can always depend on you to tell me what's going on truthfully. You've been uplifting me for over 25 years and you know the power of prayer. I love you and thank God for you.

Diane Thornton. My confidante. Sis, you always find the time to listen and care for me. You are so humble, kind and generous. You and Dallas (former Harlem Globetrotter) are special to me. You've been my friend for over 23 years. I love you and thank God for you.

1996 Allstate Bunco Club aka Bunco Bunnies. Darla Briggs, Vivian Bowman, Robin McCoy, Grace Thompson, Kim West, Carmon Thompson, and Toni Olinger. Ladies, thank you for changing the way we meet monthly to accommodate me. As a result, we're able to discuss everyone's adversities and celebrate successes. I love you all and thank God for our fellowship and the love we shared throughout the years.

Marvin Marshall. My diamond and pearl red hat diva sister and glamorous girlfriend. Sis, everything you do is Topshelf and it must be decent and in order. I love your style and the way you roll for over 21 years. Thank you for being so thoughtful and I'm grateful that you see to it that I'm glamorous too. I love you and thank God for you.

Faye Leavell. My diamond and pearl red hat diva sister and most amiable girlfriend. Cookie, you are loved by so many and I've witness first hand why. You've been there for me thru thick and thin and encouraged me to hold up my chin. Sis, you say what's on your mind, but you're always gentle and always kind. I'm so blessed we were connected through our spouses. And over the years our bond has gotten stronger. Thank you for being so good to me I love you and thank God for you.

Pastor F. Bruce & Dr. Michelle Williams and Bates Memorial Baptist Church Family. Pastor, your passion for God's Word feeds us spiritually. You've encouraged us to stay in our lane and let God guide us down the path He has given us. I must humbly say, I've done just that and received favor and blessings from the Lord. First Lady Michelle you have such a sweet spirit. I'm so blessed to have you both as our leader. Pastor, your love for Christ has caused our church family to be obedient in showing love and caring for the sick and shut in. I love you all and thank God for you.

Emmanuel A.M.E. Church, San Antonio, Texas Prayer Line Ministry. Pastor Carl Garmon Sr., First Lady Janice & Family, (Tasha, Carl Jr. & Joseph). It is because of your ministry and your faithfulness that I seek God early every morning and study His Word. I don't have enough words to say how blessed I am to be part of this ministry. There's one thing I do know, for sure, whenever I'm lifted in prayer God hears you, because something wonderful happens for me. I love you all and thank God for you.

Tracey Goodwin & Helen Swain. Sisters, you both are angels and my prayer partners. I admire your strength, your faith, your heart, and your love for God. You give generously and love unconditionally. For all these reasons, I love you and thank God for you.

Norma Jean Preston. Jean, I know we're first cousins, but you're my big sister too. Sis, you're the one God placed in my life to keep me grounded. You make sure that I receive blessings from whatever source available, and I love you for that. You're always there for me no matter what. Your love for me is genuine. Thank you for having my back Sis. I love you and thank God for you.

Sonnie Judkins. Sonnie, I know we're first cousins, but you're like a younger sister with a lot of grandkids because you are loved. You probably don't know this, but I've never forgotten how you were by my side when my first baby was born and when she passed away. I love you for that baby sis. It's been 40 years now and that love is still in my heart. I love you and thank God for you.

Falesha Price, Natosha Werner, and LaQuesha Hales. My God daughters. Ladies you all are so beautiful and special to me. I love you and thank God for you.

JaCarie Price, Kaivon Turner, and Kyeli Brandon. My Grandchildren. I'm so proud of you and I want you to always remember that you can be, have and do whatever your heart desires, if you are in the will of God. If you don't know or you want to be sure, read your bible and find your answer. I love you, and you will always and forever be special to me.

Pierre Curd and Carlos (goose) Curd. My brothers. Thank you for seeing the best in me and for always having my back. Mama and Daddy would be so proud of both of you for changing your life and worshipping God. I love you and thank God for you.

To rest of the family from the late Emma (Tee) and Jesse Curd. I love you all and I'm so grateful to have a family that loves you, lifts your spirit, encourages and not give up on you. I love each one of you and I thank God for you.

Charles H Davis (Charlie boy) aka (Pretty Ricky Fontenay). My husband. Wow! Where do I begin? Honey, you've stuck by my side through the ups and the downs. I know it has been hard not showing your emotions; wondering when I was going to get better, but God is in control, and he knows what He is doing. And even in my present state, God is still good. I'm blessed and highly favored. I'm an overcomer, and I got the victory. I was told a long time ago that I was going to win in the end. Watch and see how God is going to bless me. The best is yet to come. I appreciate you for taking care of me. I love you and thank God for you.

Raynetta Curd (Ray Ray). My dear sweet daughter. I thank God for you and I appreciate you for taking care of me. Remember to always trust and depend on God. He will never let you down, but I know you already know that. You've witnessed His goodness in my life. I love you, and thank God for you sweetie.

Ronnie McWhorter. My dear sweet son. God got you. Keep seeking Him. I will always love you, son. Keep your head up. God won't put more on you than you can handle. Stay strong. Keep the faith. I love you always no matter what and I thank God for you taking care of me.

Laura Bates and Dawn White. My Mother and Sister-n-law. I'm so grateful for everything you both have done for me in your own unique way. I love you and thank God for you.

Diamond and Pearl Divas Red Hat Society. I'm so blessed to be part of a chapter that's stunning and glamorous on the outside, as well as, on the inside. Thank you for having me in your thoughts and prayers. Thank you for your acts of kindness. I love you and thank God for you.

I would like to thank countless friends & associates for all your support for me during this journey. It doesn't go unnoticed. I'm truly blessed to have all of you in my life. I love you and thank God for you, too.

Table of Contents

Introduction

If you are waking up thinking that, 'there has got to be more to life than there is, believe that it is. But to get to that life, you're going to have to jump.'

Steve Harvey

I decided to do just that; 'JUMP,' by putting my pain, situations, setbacks, worries and concerns held on the inside of me on paper; It was therapeutic and a sense of accomplishment; furthermore, it allowed me to give birth to this unique & unforgettable book.

This is a story about a Diva; who's a social butterfly with a whole lot of swagger, faced and overcame adversities and ended up disabled and limited to a wheelchair. But through it all, she became humbled and learned how to press forward by faith. Trusting, believing and relying on God; for only He alone, has the power to change her circumstances.

My purpose is to empower, encourage, entertain and uplift your spirit. If there's anything said in this book to make it better for you, then it is a blessing to me. In fact, I hope it increases your faith, and brings healing and success to anyone that may be going through anything, that seems too impossible to handle.

In reality; when faced with what seems impossible, you think there is no way and all your hope is gone, please don't look to men for they'll let you down. God showed us how anything is possible. No matter what you've done, should have done and didn't do, he is so creative. He can do a new thing at any time and in any place, no matter what you're going through; no matter what it looks like. He does His best work in hopeless situations. He is able, and He's powerful. Keep the faith. He'll see you through. Actually, I tried Him for myself and found out that nothing is too hard for Him. Just be still and know He is God.

You're either in a storm; coming out of a storm or headed to a storm. If not, keep living, they will come for sure.

"Be kind to one another."

Ellen DeGeneres

It feels so good to be kind. It brings me joy and warms my heart. Kindness always returns. It always makes its way back to you somehow, someway from somebody.

"Be a rainbow in someone else's cloud."

Mayo Angelou

Stay Focused, Keep the Faith and Keep Going.

THE WHEELCHAIR DIVA

"IN IT TO WIN IT"

Joy and Pain

It was June 1977, when I graduated from High School. My parents wanted me to go to college. But at that time, I was unable to fulfill their dream of me going to college to become a Registered Nurse (RN), because I was 6 months pregnant. I had 3 more months to go to before having my baby; however, I always wanted a job in the medical field or the insurance industry. It didn't matter if I played a part in caring for the sick or investigated a claim to determine the extent of the insurance company's liability concerning bodily injury or property damage. It just did not matter. That was my heart desire; at that time, but not now.

I was 17 years old and really too young having responsibilities of parenting a child, but I was ready for the challenge. My parents were upset with me being pregnant; especially my father. First of all, he didn't care too much for the guy I was pregnant by because he was 10 years older than me. Likewise, he wanted the opportunity to stick his chest out and brag to his buddies and to his family members that he had a kid away in college. Anyway, I was still excited about becoming a mother.

Three months had gone by, and I had given birth to a 6 pound 8 ounce beautiful baby girl and named her Demetra Yahmelay Spencer. It was an exciting time; having a baby in the house. My cousin Sonnie was right by my side; enjoying my baby. It was as if we had a live baby doll. In fact, my brothers and parents enjoyed her as well. She was filling out fast; getting so chunky at 5 weeks old. Then one day after she had fallen asleep, I decided to go to the store. I asked Mama to check in on her. It was around 7 o'clock when I left. I thought, 'I'll go now since she was getting low on milk and pampers, so I wouldn't run out.' She was on Enfamil (milk) at the time.

Later, I returned home and Mama said, "I checked in on her, and she's still asleep," it had been over an hour or so. I peeped in on her and saw that she was sound asleep. I started thinking about having a bottle ready before she wakes up, because she sure can scream when she's hungry and I wanted to be ready. After talking to my family and getting bottles ready; it took approximately 30 minutes; I went back into the room to check in on my baby and noticed she had turned her face from sideways to face down. Back then, you would lay babies on their stomach. So, I picked her up to cuddle and hold her, and I noticed that she was not breathing.

I lost it. I screamed and hollered and said, "Something is wrong with my baby." My parents and brothers ran into the room puzzled with what I was saying. Mama called the ambulance. With the look that my parents gave each other and the tears I saw rolling down their faces, I knew then my baby had passed away. I screamed, "What's wrong with her? Why isn't she breathing? Is she dead?" I screamed and hollered for what seemed like hours. My Daddy just held on to me till the police and ambulance arrived. I was in totaled shocked; on top of that, tormented with a bunch of questions I could not get answers from the police detective, the Baby's Daddy nor our family members.

Plus, I was bombarded with questions from the neighbors and close friends. I was hearing every conversation going on all around me. I was talked about and criticize. They said, "She ain't gonna make it. She must have done something. She probably had plastic in the bed, and she was smothered." All this was being said, while my baby was still in her crib; deceased. She had to stay there until the coroner arrived to pronounce her dead.

How do you explain laying down a healthy 5 week old baby that died during her sleep? It was a devastating experience. Nothing can take away the pain or fill my baby's place in my heart. I found myself questioning the goodness of God. This is what we do; you know, when the unexpected happens to us, and we don't understand why. I cried and cried and cried. I cried so much, you would have thought somebody had beaten me in my face as puffy as my eyes were. I just couldn't get passed the fact that my baby died, and I wanted to know why. What did I do? Why was I being punished? The pain was so unbearable. All my dreams of being a mother and the plans I had for my baby girl had vanished; in an instant. And on top of that, I got to have a funeral and bury my Baby.

We received the autopsy report, and they called it 'Crib Death' because she died in her crib. Then, later called it, SIDS: Sudden Infant Death Syndrome. It's an unexplained death of a healthy baby during sleep less than a year old.

4

The Wheelchair Diva "In It to Win It"

Meantime, a week had passed and my parents had made funeral arrangements. They dressed my baby in a pretty Pink Ruffle Dress, tights, and ruffle booties. She had a Pink Ruffle Bonnet on her head with a rattle in her hand, and her daddy placed a gold ring on her finger. She looked like a beautiful Porcelain baby doll. She was placed in a small White Casket looking Bassinet. After the funeral; my Baby Daddy's Brother, Uncle John Henry was her Pallbearer. He carried the casket in his arms, got in the car and held it in his lap while traveling to Greenwood Cemetery. Then he carried it and placed it on the burial grounds. I heard them say, "Ashes to Ashes, Dust to Dust. This is the conclusion of our services, and the family will be fed at the church."

I was so numb, I couldn't even cry. The only thing I wanted to do was lay down and go to sleep. After the fellowship, that's exactly what I did. I didn't want to sleep in that room where my baby died. I stayed at my Baby Daddy's Mama's house for 2 weeks and all I did there was cry and sleep.

It was approximately 2 weeks later, when Deborah one of my classmate's, baby died the same way; hearing this overwhelmed me. I had to go visit and bond with her. I was able to share my grief with someone who understood my pain. The following week later; Sherry, another one of our classmate's baby died of SIDS as well. I was able to share my feelings with both classmates who had similar losses. It was comforting and healing for me to connect with them, because we all were grieving the loss of a baby.

However, the grieving process still took a while longer than normal. In fact, I was told that I was experiencing 'Complicated Grief.' It can come from a sudden death of a loved one or a mother mourning the death of her child. A counselor explained to me that individuals who have lost a loved one suddenly or in a tragic accident are at a higher risk of developing complicated grief. Complicated grief can last for months or years. I didn't have any energy whatsoever. Nothing motivated me. I felt numb, and had sorrowful feelings; constantly longing for my baby.

When we get expose to difficulties, it's the only way for our faith in God to grow. I started praising and praying for strength to endure this pain I'd been experiencing. It took me about a year to get it together, but finally I started going back to church surrounding myself around love ones. Later, I gave my hand to God. And through all my trials and tribulations, I found out that God is my joy in time of sorrow. He's been my all in all. I will never let go of his hand.

It was approximately 2 years later, I went to insurance school and gave birth to another beautiful bouncing baby girl; Raynetta Nicole Curd. Then 3 years later, I married at 24 and had my son; Ronnie Maurice McWhorter while working in the medical field, and I later received my Independent Insurance Adjuster License.

Stay focused; Keep the Faith, and Keep Going.

The Journey

'Do what you got to do, to do what you want to do.'

Denzel Washington

It just didn't work out. I was 27, divorced with 2 kids and trying to make ends meet. "Sometimes it's hard being a woman having to submit to a man." I told this to an older gentleman and a real good friend of mine, whose about 20 years older than me. And he said to me, "Girl, you built like a brick house; you got a big old booty too. Dammit girl, you got a bad ass body any man would pay for. You pretty and you smart. And you know what else? You got a gold mine between your legs. Plus, you can cook." He went on to say, "You should never be broke another day in your life, if you do it right and use it right." And then he ended up saying, "You should use what you got to get what you want."

I know I was listening to a dirty old man; but at this stage in the game, I was tired of struggling and ready to live a glamorous life while having fun doing it. I went into beast mode. I decided to do just what he said and put it to the test;

I thought. It's not my job to fix a man, but I can feed him, please him and receive daily benefits, and that's what this Diva did. I didn't make any rules. I just went with the flow and put on captivating performances with vivid imaginations.

My first client was a business man with a side hustle. He was really a gangster on the side; he was shrewd, but we'd known each other for years. We never messed around, but always flirted with each other. He's definitely a bad boy, stood about 6 ft., built like a capital "Y", tight butt, fine with smooth brown skin, pretty teeth, just drop dead good-looking, with dimples. He had a nice fade, always sharp, always smelling good and had a beautiful smile. He drove a nice Caddy, and he was about to be all mines. I thought, 'Let me see what he's got going on.' We talked, and he planned to take me out to dinner and a movie.

On the other hand; on this particular day, I decided that I was going to be a 'star' in my own show. I was going to be a little naughty, while cooking his favorite meal in the Sexist Lingerie I had in my closet with my Stilettoes on. He was picking me up at 7. The doorbell ranged. I opened it. He stepped in the door; while looking at me, and he dropped to his knees acting crazy. We're both laughing, while he's getting up. He said, "This is quite a surprise." I started walking around switching from side to side; gyrating my body with sounds of Wendell B playing in the back ground.

I was having complete control; playing by my own rules, being sensual, kind spoken and smelling good. After having a few cocktails, we ate the dinner I'd prepared for us. Afterwards, he helped me clean up the kitchen. We continued drinking Woodford Reserve, smoking plenty of weed while kissing and slow dancing. I'd noticed that he was getting tickled, pulled back from me and said, "Baby you 'shol do look good, but you got your shoes on the wrong feet." We laughed until we cried, and what a night to remember. You couldn't tell me anything. I knew I was looking good being a sex kitten. We had too much fun. He really spoiled me. Oh, what a night.

Truthfully, I didn't have too many other men lined up liked I'd planned. Because he made sure I lived like a queen, and had my back no matter what; I didn't want for nothing. He even had me carrying a 9mm in my designer bag that he brought me. He said, "Keep it in your purse at all times for protection. You live alone with these kids, and you need a piece of steel in your possession when I'm not around." Wow, what you can say about that?

You got to know what you want out of life, and you cannot be afraid to show it and look fabulous doing it. Just be who you are. This went on for 7 years. I became very creative; putting on stellar performances. He paid very well. I had an excellent compensation package and even travelled with him on business trips. After a while, he became jealous and started stalking me. I realized then that I needed to transition from being the Tycoon's diva. I had to go gangster on him. Remember that 9 mm he gave me for protection? After I got away from him and being pinned up against the wall, I drew that 9 mm out on him and got my respect.

I was intrigued with bad boys, and I had quite a few back in the day. In fact, along with the Shrewd Business man, there was another Gangster, Hustler, Baller, Drug Dealer, Dentist, Professor, Soldier, Deacon, and even a Stripper (**Dirty Dancer**). He would make love to you without even touching you. Hell, I often thought about having a 'Stripper house.' You know like 'Magic Mike XXL.' Oh my goodness! I'm having a flashback. Remember the scene when Channel Tatum & Twitch (Ellen DeGeneres, DJ) stripped. MY! MY! MY! Can you imagine dollar bills raining down in every room of your house, and your guest having their wildest fantasies come true?

There it goes again; having a creative mind. Really, this is completely, outrageously fun for me. And if you are there making it rain; it's clear to me, it's enjoyment for you too. But wait a minute! They don't have anything on my fine ass husband, '**Pretty Ricky Fonteynay**!' You see, I've given my husband a stage name. Well let me clarify; the husband number 3, I'm presently married to.

Actually, I have enjoyed and learned something from all of them. They made me into the diva I am today. With my creative mind, I made things happen and got things done. I did what I thought was best at that particular time. Surely, you can have the right motive, but end up doing the wrong thing. Eventually; find yourself being in front of a judge, answering questions for the way you handle things. Your heart can be right, but the way you handle the situation can be wrong. Just face it and own up to whatever you've done;

13

I did.

We all stumble in many ways. According to James 3:2 (CEV), "All of us do many wrong things." So stop beating yourself up and run towards Jesus. Receive His grace and mercy. He's already forgiven you. Now, forgive yourself.

I no longer wanted this lifestyle. I felt like I was missing something anyway. These fantasies that I created showed me that I was empty on the inside. I got to think more of myself than wasting my life being something that I'm not. I needed discipline. I needed to learn how to be patient and wait on what I wanted. No more, 'I got to have it right now.' No more manipulation. I wanted to have someone in my life to love me just the way I am. I'm enough just the way I am. I want a man to see my heart, my loyalty, my love, and not some fantasy; well maybe sometimes. Please don't get me wrong, I really enjoyed it while it lasted. I'm here to please.

Honestly, I wanted to be valued. I just wanted to settle down and become a virtuous woman. I wanted to be with someone who would follow God and serve him. We serve Him with our whole heart and soul. We seek after Him and follow His ways. We trust Him and stand on His word. God is faithful, powerful, and He is in charge.

But, do you know what I found out about myself? There's a warrior deep down on the inside of me. Up till now, he's never forgotten about my first performance after all these years. And still today, when I run into him, (the shrewd business man; hustler/ gangster), he laughs at me and tells me, 'If I needed him for anything, he is there for me.' Really! If it was left up to him, I would've received a star on the Hollywood walk of fame with all the acts I put on. I surprised myself being so artistic.

Inside this book, you will understand why this Diva became humble and stayed in her lane. You will learn that it takes courage to be different. It takes courage to win.

However; this Diva made some mistakes in life, but she honestly repented and has done her best to do the right thing since then. So, please, don't judge. Let's not forget, that none of us is perfect. We've all made some mistakes. We all have areas in which we need to improve. Now, let go of the guilt and shame. Release it into the hands of the Almighty God. He has forgiven you. Forgive yourself.

More importantly, you will realize that God uses difficulties to move us towards our destiny. You grow in the tough times. It's during the tough times that we find out what we are really made of. Most of all, we need to cooperate with God in order to see the finish works of Jesus recognizable in our life. So, this Diva started relying on God, changed her way of thinking and developed a renewed mind.

This Diva must put her '**Big Girl Panties'** on to face these challenges that have come upon her. What's more, you will identify that this '*social butterfly'* had a whole lot of swagger before she became a Diva in a wheelchair.

On this journey, she's seeking total victory, restoration, deliverance, healing, abundance and prosperity. It's time to move forward by faith. God is in control. He's ordering and directing her steps, and she needs to move at His pace.

** Even if you stumble and fall, just get back up and keep walking with Jesus. He's moving you in the direction He wants you to go. At least you are moving forward.

Stay focused; Keep the Faith, and Keep Going.

I Am Somebody

For so long, I hid my pain of being told by a boss that I had '***bad grammar.***' This seed of negativity formed doubt, stress and fear inside me; including, affecting my ability of speaking publicly. Putting on presentations was out of the question. I was so afraid that I would freeze up, start stuttering, break out in a sweat and that my blood pressure would go up. It just made me sick. In fact, I had clear understanding on how to do certain assignments, but would shy away from training others.

Likewise, I avoided speaking up, brainstorming and collaborating with the Executive team on ways to solve problems anticipated on a new project, before we got it up and running. Instead, my mind was focused on what '*somebody said about me.*' The truth is, 'What do I say about me?' I'm a person of integrity, with a creative mind and kind to others who is unique and wonderfully made by God. I have skills and talents inside me that I didn't even know I had; which now, I'm giving birth to. For that reason, I cannot continue to let what other people think or say about me, affect me.

Also, I cannot allow someone else's insecurities affect me any longer. I've cried my last tear. Haters will hate. They saw something in me that made them jealous and furious with me. It's obvious; they wanted what I had, which comes natural for me. Really, they were afraid I was going to get something they wanted. Whatever the case, the devil had to do something. And the only thing he could come up with was to voice his opinion about my grammar.

But guess what; here I go again, being brought down on my knees. I must remember that the Lord is on my side. I know how to praise and pray my way through. This weapon thrown against me is not going to prosper; I must be still. Wait and see.

Yes, I spoke and explained things the way I understood them to be. However, their negativity hurt my feelings; bad. It made me question my own capabilities and shut me down. I may not be an English scholar, but I'm very clear and did get my point across. I had to decide whose voice I was going to listen to, and whose opinion about me was I going to believe, God or man?

The Wheelchair Diva "In It to Win It"

**THE WORD OF GOD IS MY WEAPON

**THE WORD OF GOD IS POWERFUL; IT CHANGES THINGS

The bible says in Hebrews 13:6 (ESV), ".....The Lord is my helper; I will not fear; what can man do to me?"

** They meant it for evil, but God worked it out for my good.

Let me explain. One day at work, I spoke with the media about a medical claim that was processed and adjusted per the patient's insurance policy. The disgruntle insured patient was upset about the way the claim was processed, that he made accusations of filing a bad faith claim. But instead of coming to us, he went to the media to be heard all because his out of pocket expenses were more than what the insurance company paid towards his claim. After reviewing his policy, it was very clear to me that he did not understand his insurance coverages.

Therefore, I had to explain to the insured patient, the media, the VP of Claims operations, along with the management team on how this claim was processed line by line. Yes, me! The so called, 'bad grammar' adjuster, broke it down for them all and made it so simple that a nine year old could understand. As a result, not only did he apologize, but I was acknowledged for a job '**Well done,'** by the executive team, which included, a promotion and later on a bonus.

Ain't God good? **WON'T HE DO IT FOR YOU?**

Psalms 118:6 (GNB), "The Lord is with me, I will not be afraid; what can anyone do to me?"

Proverbs 8:35 (NLT), "For whoever finds me finds life and receives favor from the Lord."

We all have experienced the favor of God in our lives. It's because of the love He has for us, that we receive His favor. Truthfully, we don't have to do anything to deserve this favor. Still, we should stay connected to God by communicating daily through prayer, by our continuous praise & worship and by studying His Word.

Proverbs 16:7 (MSG), "When God approves of your life, even your enemies will end up shaking your hand."

In other words; when our ways pleases God, God will

do some wonderful things in our lives. He will take our enemies and make them to be at peace with us. You can even turn your enemies into friends, especially when they see godly character operating in our lives.

Still, pray for the favor of God. He will open up doors for you, the right people will come into your life, and you will discover His favor operating in unexpected places. It is because of His favor that things worked out for my good.

**Don't let anybody stop you from being all God created you to be. In fact; my grammar just wasn't up to his standards, but it was good enough to save the company from an embarrassing lawsuit or a nuisance settlement. You see, nothing can happen that you and God cannot handle together.

**Evil plus God = good; whenever evil shows up and God is in the equation, good comes out of it.

Now at 45 years old, I'd been married to my second husband for 7 years when he abandoned me after I had lost my daycare. I wanted to start my own business which we both agreed that it was the right time. So, I decided to give a 2 week notice to terminate my 6 year employment with

Sonja P. Davis

AIG Specialty Auto Insurance Company.

Everything was going great for us, until one day I had a meeting at 4C's and my workers decided to leave a baby unattended on the floor, while outback watching the other kids playing and smoking weed. A parent caught them outback and told his wife about it. She removed their children without my knowledge, and had a state worker at my door. I was able to obtain my license, but I had to fire my workers. Now, there were no kids to care for. Because I kept a family of children, you know how that goes. Everybody was pissed off. And I can't blame them, I just didn't have the energy to recruit other children to keep it going. However, I often wonder how the children are doing and I pray all is well with them.

This was hard for us as my income was a major part of paying the household expenses. So, the pressure caused my husband to step out of our marriage. Later, I caught him wining and dining with some other 'scallywag.' I was so heart broken.

**"Then Jesus said, Come to me, all of you who are weary and carry heavy burdens, and I will give you rest."

The Wheelchair Diva "In It to Win It"

This is found in Matthew 11:28 (NLT).

So here I was again Lord having to drop to my knees in pain because of my husband's abandonment, the loss of my daycare, and I got served foreclosure papers along with being audited by the IRS. "Father, please come down here to see about me. I don't mind waiting on you. I know that you're able to get me through this, you've done it before and I know you can do it again."

Plus, I truly loved that man. I wasn't going to be without an income for long. It was a little setback. I knew how to make ends meet. I just needed him to be by myside. I couldn't eat, I couldn't sleep, and I wished I didn't love him so much because this felt like a loved one had died, after getting a divorce. I cried and cried and cried. Then later my faith grew after continuous prayer and praising. Somehow; in some way, I regained strength. I started getting stronger and stronger. My sunshine had come on a cloudy day. It was my due season. I knew it was. It had to have been, because I was still in my right mind. I'm so proud of me keeping it all together. I could have lost my mind.

But God is my refuge, and He is my strength. He is

my help in times of trouble. (Psalms 46:1) He dried my tears and He drove all my fears away. How can you not serve a God that is so faithful? That's kind and compassionate and loves you unconditionally.

Later, God did bless me with another job as a Senior Workers Compensation Insurance Adjuster for AP Capital. Things had gotten better, so much better. Thank you, Lord.

**You don't have to struggle for other people's approval when you know you're loved and accepted by God.

Now, stop worrying about what people think about you. God is not going to bless you on how people think. Don't allow negative thoughts take up space in your mind. Be still and know that he is God. He is greater than any situation you face. So don't quit. Stay in the race.

So, this is only a small part of my story, and I pray it inspired and blessed you. It's simply been a breakthrough for me. As you read this book, I hope it lends a hand in seeking God for whatever situation, issue or circumstance you face; as well as, you receiving the breakthrough that you need.

I pray this book gives hopefulness through your day

and joy on tomorrow. Being so captivating, that it raises your spirits and has you run towards Jesus worshipping Him and giving Him all the glory; the entire honor and all of the praise which He deserves; because He's worthy.

Father God, I thank you and bless you for what you're doing and what you've already done. Thank you for another opportunity to help a brother or sister who may be struggling and don't know which way to turn. I offer them you, and only you. Honestly, there is no other. Truly, there are benefits in trusting and serving you...In Jesus name. Amen.

"But in that coming day, no weapon turned against you will succeed. You will silence every voice raised up to accuse you. These benefits are enjoyed by the servants of the Lord; their vindication will come from me. I, the Lord, have spoken!" (Isaiah 54:17, NLT)

Stay focused; Keep the Faith, and Keep Going.

Up Close and Personal / My Path / My Lane

"You are the one who put me together inside my mother's body, and I praise you because of the wonderful way you created me. Everything you do is marvelous!" (Psalms 139:13-14 CEV)

Presently at age 57, this Diva had been married 3 three times. She re-married her third husband, raised 2 kids and has 3 grandchildren. She worked in the Insurance industry for 30 years and became an outstanding Independent Insurance Adjuster with these companies, Humana, Blue Cross Blue Shield, Aetna, Healthcare Recoveries Inc., York Insurance, AP Capital, Allstate and AIG. Also, worked 5 years as a co-manager for one of the largest grocery retail food chain, Kroger.

Formerly, Vice President of Lace Social Club, she was also a member of the Ebonaise Social and Civic Club which sponsored the Ebony Fashion Show at the Memorial Auditorium here in Louisville, Kentucky. Presently, she is a member of the Red Hat Society Diamond and Pearl Divas; including being a member of the Bunco club, with the

Sonja P. Davis

Allstate Insurance Adjusters, since 1996.

Moreover, this diva is quite stunning and glamorous. She wore exquisite clothing that stood out amongst the rest. Besides, her presentation from head to toe is a gift to you. She would often say, "Dress like you want to be addressed. Let people see that you are blessed." Actually, this came from her mother. As a child, her mother loved her and dressed her like a little princess. She grew up blessed feeling special with all her needs met. Her mother's presentation was a gift to her, by the way she honors God with her smile and by the attire she would wear for worship. Oh how adorable; just simply gorgeous. She would always say, "God deserves our very best."

Her smile is her style. It warms your heart and stimulates conversations. People are drawn to her like a magnet. The energy she gives off uplifts your spirit. Whenever you're feeling down and in her presence, nothing seems to bother you as much. Your frown turns into a smile. She's very positive.

Plus, she's a wife, mother, grandmother, godmother, sister, cousin, niece, auntie and a treasured friend. Her family truly loves and adores her. She has the ability to bring the best out of you. Her husband often says, "You better not leave me. I need you in my life. We are better together than we are apart." Her girlfriends call her 'sister,' because she's so loyal, kind, fun, compassionate, sympathetic, generous; and most of all, an excellent cook. Her brothers look to her as 'Mama.' She loves decorating, traveling, shopping and finding bargains. She calls it fun and energizing.

Furthermore, she is an educated woman and a lifelong learner. She enjoys reading and loves being taught. And by the way, she has earned an MBA from Ottawa University. She often drank 'Moscato Wine' and smoked plenty of 'Weed' after having several failed marriages and trying to get her through school. She probably could have smoked 'Snoop Dog' under the table. Hold up! Don't judge! Not a perfect Diva. It was hard working and going to school trying to get a degree. But wait a minute! Who she fooling? It was God's grace and His mercy that got her through, for they are new every morning. (Lamentations 3:22-23).

Also she drove luxury cars; the latest, a 2008 Jaguar XJ Vanden Plas. She is very creative, and has an eye for beauty and flair; let say, a 'touch of class.' She was once featured on Bob Sokoler; co-host of WHAS-TV's 'Louisville Tonight Live' segment called 'The Wild Thing' for including animal print in her beautiful home decor. Bob was showcasing how black residents live in the West End of Louisville, KY (1998-1999). Not all of us are trifling. We like nice things too! Thank you, Anita for making this possible.

She enjoys horse racing, likes things that go fast, that are strong, rough, and tough like a Stallion, Football Player, Basketball Player and even a Boxer. She is intrigued with bad boys. She's loyal, creative, calculating, a go getter, a ride or die type chick, a survivor, a cheerleader, a problem solver, a model, a dancer, generous, fun and a Christian.

More importantly; the best thing about this Diva is, she's very inspirational and an encourager. Her faith in God helps pull you through. She's a voice of love and shows it. She has the gift of generosity and hospitality; she's great at it and can back it up.

In fact, it was time to celebrate the Senior Pastor of Bates Memorial Baptist church. It was Pastor F Bruce

The Wheelchair Diva "In It to Win It"

William's Anniversary. It was a special time where you could encourage him and show your appreciation for him feeding us spiritually. This diva wanted to express and demonstrate how blessed she was in having him as our leader, and wanted him to know that he was loved and cared for. Truthfully, he's very blessed. She has Wayne Brown, owner of Suit Man Custom Clothiers; a very dear friend and a Custom Tailor out of Cincinnati, Ohio, to tailor a suit for Pastor Williams. We wanted Pastor Williams to look like he's blessed. We wanted him to look sharp in his Tailored Made Suits when he went out of town on special engagements. Therefore, Wayne custom-made several suits to show Pastor Williams how much we cared and truly appreciated him.

For that reason; if you attend church, encourage your Pastor, Reverend, Minister, Bishop, Priest, Apostle, Elder, Clergy or your overseer; whoever is the leader of your church and is sent by God. Pray for him or her. Keep them uplifted. Express to them that you care for them and show love and respect their mate. I know that's ashame, but we have to throw that in there, because it's the truth. Therefore,

I need to acknowledge our dear, sweet First Lady, Dr. Michelle Williams. Thank you for being an example of a virtuous woman, kind, compassionate and supportive. May God continue to bless you.

**You'll never know how successful you can be until you get rid of the things that slow you down and trip you up. Please, don't give up on God. Don't just pray. Believe. Keep the faith.

**Bishop T.D. Jakes says, "If I can kill it in my head. I can kill it in my life. Every time you get dirt thrown on you, throw it behind you. Every time you throw it behind you, God is raising you up." Bishop Jakes went on to say, "He is a loyal person." So am I and generous too. "Be that type of guy; a limited resource person. I have to watch giving out my high octane love to that low octane engine. My love is too rich to plant it in poor soil. I'm willing to do too much for you, than to do it for just anybody. I go too far, before I realize that I've done planted good seed in bad soil. Then my feelings get hurt. My confidence gets low. I give too much to too little. It's not your fault; it's mine, for not valuing my deposits."

The Wheelchair Diva "In It to Win It"

**You got to know who you are. When you know whose you are, don't ever forget who you are. Stay true to yourself.

**Never pay back evil with more evil. Do all you can to live in peace with everyone! Never take revenge, leave that to God. For the bible says, "I will take revenge; I will pay them back, says the Lord." (Romans 12:17-19 NLT.)

Stay focused; Keep the Faith, and Keep Going

Sonja P. Davis

I Can't Handle This

"This is my command; be strong and courageous! Do not be afraid or discouraged. For the Lord your God is with you wherever you go." (Joshua 1:9, NLT)

God knew that the assignment He called Joshua to do was more than he could handle.

You're usually in a storm, coming out of a storm or heading into a storm.

"So encourage each other and build each other up, just as you are already doing." (1 Thesalonians 5:11, NLT)

I don't understand it. I didn't know what was wrong. I had a few back surgeries and the latest one was a back fusion from L1 to S1 that I had recovered from. It just didn't make since. I began to struggle getting up from sitting down; pulling up from squatting; walking a short distance; going up and down stairs; and lifting my arms to comb my hair. I knew it couldn't be from my back; but maybe, it is.

Then it happened, when I woke up one morning; I

was unable to walk. There I went again; brought back down on my knees. I knew I had to praise and pray my way through. I cried and I prayed, "Lord do it. Do it for me, right now. I know you're able. I'm calling on you, Jesus."

"Father, I need to release into your hands the things I don't understand. Forgive me for worrying, as I walk with you through this difficult situation. I have no doubt in my mind that, you Lord, can help me. I'm down here waiting on you. And by the way, troubles don't last always. So, whatever I'm going through is only temporary."

Stay focused; Keep the Faith, and Keep Going

The Wheelchair Diva "In It to Win It"

Running To You

(Lyrics from my heart)

Can't take it

Can't make it, without you

What do I do?

What shall I do?

Must run to you

Father, oh Father, I can't handle this situation that has come

upon me.

What am I supposed to do?

But, run to you

Have to run to you.

What else is there to do?

Just don't know what to do

But keep running to you

Keep running. Don't stop running

Keep running. Can't stop running

Sonja P. Davis

Keep running. Won't stop running

Lord you have power to step into my situation
My soul has been anchored with you
Everything you do is simply marvelous
The only thing to do is run towards you.
Keep running, keep on running

I keep stumbling & falling, but still
Keep running. Don't stop, keep on running

"But Jesus, I stopped to look back at my past to fix it. You said learn from it and let it go. You taught me how to take my past and find my path."
Keep running. Can't stop, keep on running

"Oh Father, I need some fresh anointing to overcome these difficulties I face. Even with my unanswered questions, I choose to trust you and run to you."
Keep running. Won't stop, Got to keep on running

The Wheelchair Diva "In It to Win It"

"You can make my wrongs right. You can turn my messes into miracles."
Don't stop, Can't stop, and won't stop running. Got to keep on running

"I believe in a God who loves performing the impossible. I'm going to be still and know who you are."
Don't stop, Can't stop, and won't stop running. Got to keep on running

"Jesus, I surrender all of me, as I run to you. Thank you for leading me and guiding me into the palm of your hands."
Don't stop, Can't stop, and won't stop running. Got to keep on running

"Lord, now that I'm in your presence, things are better all around me. I've been purified and strengthen.
Thank you for working things out for my good and for your glory."
Can't stop, and won't stop running
Got to keep on running

Can't stop, and won't stop

Got to keep on running to you

**Put God first. Worship Him for who He is. Chase after Him.

**Press on towards Him. Keep running to Him. His blessings will come.

**To avoid getting tripped up, don't look back at your past. You can't change it. But you can run toward Jesus and learn from it.

Stay focused; Keep the Faith, and Keep Going.

Help Me

"O Lord my God, I cried to you for help, and you restored my health." (Psalm 30:2, NLT).

God is definitely up to something. He is uniquely preparing me to do something special for His Kingdom. I need to have faith for what I don't know. Now it's time to go to the doctor to find out exactly what's going on with me. After being cleared from my back surgeon to rule-out anything to do with my back, I was referred to *Dr. Joseph Oropilla, Neurologist with Kentucky One Health Neurology Associates*. He was determined to find out what caused me not to walk. So, he ordered an emergency MRI of the spinal cord to rule-out paralysis from a spinal cord injury. Then he performed an EMG and ran several blood tests, and diagnosed me with having 'Myopathy,' which means muscle disease. He wanted me to get a second opinion so I was referred to U of L Physicians Neurologist; Dr. Martin Brown. He diagnosed me, as having, a muscle disease, as well and called it "*Myositis.*" He went on to say that, "Myositis describes inflammation or swelling of the muscle tissue.

General muscle inflammation can occur after exercise or taking certain medication, or it can be from a chronic inflammatory muscle disorder like 'polymyositis.'"

In fact; based on my symptoms, he named it '*Polymyositis*' because my muscle weakness is proximal in many areas close to my body. According to The Myositis Association (TMA), Polymyositis is a disease that causes inflammation and weakness of your muscles. It can also affect your skin tissues. Polymyositis is also known as idiopathic inflammatory myopathy. It is often associated with diseases in which the body attacks its own cells (autoimmune diseases). The cause of polymyositis is not known. The disease is common in adults. It's more common in women.

To diagnose polymyositis, your health care provider will take your medical history and do a physical exam. My symptoms were weakness in my neck, shoulders, upper arms, hip and thighs. I had difficulty rising from a seated position, climbing stairs, lifting things, reaching overhead, swallowing, fatigue and sore muscles.

Also, various tests may be done, including: Blood

tests, MRI and EMG. EMG (electromyography) this test is done to check electrical activity of the muscle, and a muscle biopsy; which a sample of muscle tissue is examined to check for an underlining condition such as cancer.

It has been said that there is no cure for polymyositis, but treatment can improve muscle strength and function. The earlier treatment is started, the more effective it is. For treatment, I received Prednisone, (a corticosteroid which helped with inflammation). Physical and Occupational Therapy is part of your treatment as well.

After having all these tests ran, I was admitted in U of L Hospital to start taking steroids intravenously to attack the muscle disease and to wait for test results on the muscle biopsy from Vanderbilt University. Ten days had passed and no signs of cancer found. "Hallelujah! Thank you Jesus!"

However, the test confirmed the diagnosis of *Polymyositis.* Now it's time to go to Frazier Rehab for inpatient Physical Therapy. At this facility, they would help strengthen my muscles. And they have equipment that would assist me in my ability to walk. I stayed there for 6 weeks, which did improve my mobility. But still, I'm not walking.

Therefore, Physical Therapy continued at Frazier Rehab at one of their outpatient facilities. However, was still taking steroids; which is something else I didn't want to do, because they blow you up and causes weight gain. But if I wanted to get well, I had to. I really didn't want to, but I had to. If I wanted this muscle disease to leave my body, I had to think again.

Well, 8 months had gone by of being in outpatient rehab. I was not progressing. I was at a standstill; and guess what, was still not walking. I'd been referred back to the Frazier Rehab doctor; Dr. Sarah Wagers and to my Neurologist, Dr. Martin Brown. I was seeing them occasionally anyway throughout my therapy to have lab work done. It was necessary to have Labs ran every 8 weeks, because steroids can cause other medical problems such as: Diabetes, Eye problems, Hypertension and Obesity, just to name a few.

Wow Polymyositis! This was actually what I was experiencing; Why me? This diva had to continue being in a wheelchair. I couldn't do it. I didn't want to, but I had no other choice. I had to. Look closely; and chances are, you'd see God.

Then one day, my girlfriend Faye called me. Her husband passed away. Now, I had a decision to make; although, she told me not to worry about coming over and attending anything. She knew my heart was with her. On many occasions, I'd been there for all my girlfriends. I had to go to my girlfriend husband's funeral. In fact, he was also my husband's best friend. Fred, there will never be another one like you. He was one sharp brother.

In that moment, I made the decision to accept what had happened to me and went on to the funeral. My presence lifted her spirit; which in turn, blessed me as well. Although; it sadden others to see me this way, cause they knew how I rolled. However; the truth was, this was a breakthrough for me. From that day, I decided to put my pain to paper. And with a leap of faith, I jumped, began writing my journey of being in a wheelchair and birthed, 'The Wheelchair Diva.'

I knew I must bring awareness to this disease and become a Patient Advocate. I wanted to be part of the solution, instead of complaining about the problem. I can't spend all my time trying to figure out why. Why did I develop this muscle disease? But, I did know that God was in control, and I was where He wanted me to be. In fact; somehow, someway, I was going to get through this even if I had to go down fighting.

Whatever you're going through, don't stay down; rise up. You got this with determination and positivity.

Besides; Muhammed Ali said, "The ground is no place for a champion. If you look up, you can get up." The champ went on to say, "There are no pleasures in a fight, but some of my fights have been a pleasure to win."

Furthermore, how can I talk about how good God is, if I've never been through nothing? Truthfully; how can I say He's a healer, if I've never been sick? It's good that I been afflicted. If I had not been afflicted, I would never know the power of God.

In fact, I do know the power of God. Nothing I've been through has been more traumatic than the loss of my baby girl, and I got through that by giving God my hand. And I've never let go.

In order to have a remarkable recovery, you have to

be content in whatever state you're in. You have to have a stable mind. Mental stability aids in your recovery. You have to ask God for wisdom, knowledge and understanding to accept what happened. You've got to humble yourself and give God the praise. You can't be healed until you deal with the problem. Don't leave God out of any circumstances you face.

"Father God, thank you for being with me. I don't have to be alone with these difficulties I face. I must keep in mind and believe that I have what it takes to get through this experience."

** When you get through your experience, look back and thank God for the things He brought you through and taught you along the way.

**The Bible says in Mark 9:23 (NLT), "Anything is possible if a person believes." In every situation, I do believe. And by believing in the power of God, I have nothing to lose but everything to gain. The truth is I don't mind waiting on the Lord.

God, what you promised I believe, and it will come

to pass. Nothing can happen that you and I cannot handle together.

Stay focused; Keep the Faith, and Keep Going

It Takes Faith

"So faith comes from hearing that is, hearing the Good News about Christ." (Romans 10:17, NLT)

"Without faith no one can please God. Whoever comes to God must believe that he is real and he rewards those who sincerely try to find him." (Hebrews 11:6, ERV).

"Don't you remember that our ancestor Abraham was shown to be right with God by his actions when he offered his son Isaac on the altar? You see his faith and his actions worked together. His actions made his faith complete. And so it happened just as the Scriptures said, Abraham believed God, and God counted him as righteous because of his faith." He was even called a friend of God. So you see, we are shown to be right with God by what we do, not by faith alone. "Just as the body is dead without breath, so also faith is dead without good works." (James 2:21-24, 26 NLT).

Have faith and believe in the Word of God. It has power. We have the authority and power by faith to speak things into existence.

Faith is the confidence that what we hope for will actually happen. I am the healed. This disease must leave my body and never come back again. I will walk again, and I'll dance again. I believe in the finish works of Jesus.

Faith believes before you see it. Even if you don't see a way, know that the Lord can make a way. So, hold on to your faith, believe in the Word of God and have no doubt.

God is restoring health back into me. I'll become what I believe; more than a conqueror and well able to succeed. 'Polymyositis,' you are defeated. You can't stay here. You are coming down. I'm getting better and better in every way, every day.

**You cannot speak negative and expect positive results. You come this far by faith; leaning and depending on the Lord.

**God didn't bring me this far to leave me, nor you. So I encourage you to believe in yourself. You can make it, no matter how deep your valley may be in your life. Never give up. You're never alone in your voyage of faith. Surrender your crisis, concerns or circumstances; give them over to God. He got you. Reach out, stretch and touch the hem of His garment. You'll be made whole. Believe and receive God's supernatural miracle working power released in your life.

We must not forget that our God is powerful. And where do you think we get power from? Let us not forget that we receive power from God. In fact, He's so awesome and powerful that His Holy Spirit empowers us with what we need in order to carry out His plans He has for us.

Stay focused; Keep the Faith, and Keep Going

Tell It Like It Is

Oprah Winfrey once said, "***Make every moment teachable.***"

I have no doubt that God has a good plan for my life. He uniquely prepared me to be in this wheelchair. It is no accident that I'm here. I wouldn't be here unless He had a purpose for it. I have to be satisfied with where I am right now. Lord, open my eyes to see how I can serve you right where I am. I've been planted, and I'm coming up. As I renew my mind with the Word of God, He is transforming me. This transformation won't have me looking the same nor being the same.

Instead of complaining and expecting defeat, don't lose sleep or get discourage. God is turning every stumbling block into a stepping stone. He is with you and for you. If you get knocked down, you'll get back up again. No matter what comes against you. Totally believe God.

**Become a problem solver. Help someone else who may be going through something similar.

53

Sonja P. Davis

*"**Be a rainbow in somebody's cloud**."* Dr. Mayo Angelou

My situation may be taking longer than I thought, but that's okay. According to Jeremiah 29:11-13 (NIV), "For I know the plans I have for you declares the Lord. Plans to prosper you and not to harm you, plans to give you hope and a future. Then you will call on me and come and pray to me, and I will listen to you. You will seek me and find me, when you seek me with all your heart."

While God is working with me in a place I don't want to be, he's setting something up over in another place to bless others through me; which is my divine assignment. God is going to show me His favor and His power in my life like I've never seen before. I am in the palm of His hands. He is in control. He is so amazing.

Also the Bible says in Jeremiah 32:27 (NKJV), "Behold, I am the Lord, the God of all flesh. Is there anything too hard for me?"

Father God, when you bring me out of this, everybody around me is going to have no doubt that, 'nothing is too hard for you.' For that reason, you might as well get ready because the God I serve is awesome. Cry out to Him. Go to Him. Tell Him exactly how you feel. He's never surprised by or even gets upset by any of your emotions. You cannot expect anybody else to meet a need that only God can fulfill.

Stay focused; Keep the Faith, and Keep Going

But God

Then Jesus said to the disciples in Mark 11:22-24 (NLT), "Have faith in God. I tell you the truth, you can say to this mountain, May you be lifted up and thrown into the sea, and it will happen. But you must really believe it will happen and have no doubt in your heart. I tell you, you can pray for anything, and if you believe that you've received it, it will be yours."

You got to open your mouth and speak to that mountain. Tell that mountain its coming down. Therefore; sickness, debt, fear, loneliness and depression, I may be down now but I am not staying down. I'm coming up. I will rise again. Whatever your mountain, you got the authority to speak to it. Tell it to come down; it doesn't have any place here. In the name of Jesus!

Wait a minute! But God sometimes inconveniences us to help somebody else who may be going through something similar. So, quit complaining. Father, I don't understand it. Why did this happen to me? This doesn't make sense to me. Nevertheless; I believe, I will understand it better by and by.

This difficulty looked like a setback, but God ordered it, to use it, to move me forward, to do the impossible and to help build my faith. Really, it's a minor setback for a major comeback. I'm on my road to recovery. God is giving me beauty for my ashes. God is in control of each and everything in our lives.

You see this diva rides to the beat of her own drum: 'Once a Diva, always a Diva.' "I can't be something that I'm not, and I want wear a mask." You're right about that Gladys. She went from stilettoes to non-slip footies. Besides, when she rises up, she won't slip and fall. She went from wearing elegant sophisticated clothing, to loose, comfortable and beautiful Kaftans. Kaftans have their own style and flair. Wear them and feel like a queen. It brings out the Royal Goddess in you.

She went from driving a Jaguar, to rolling in what she now calls her chariot, '*the wheelchair*.' It doesn't matter; just be you. You don't have to compete with other people. What God allowed is unique to me. God gave me the grace to face this challenge of being in a wheelchair. I have to be content in whatever state I'm in. I know what it's like being up, and I know what it's like being down. A whole lot of people couldn't handle this being in a wheelchair.

This little light of mine, I'm going to let it shine. Let it shine, let it shine, let it shine.

Stay focused; Keep the Faith, and Keep Going

Won't He Do It

Submitted facts to prove this to candid people

He is; at this time, is able;

Ephesians 3:20-21 (MSG), "God can do anything; you know, far more than you could ever imagine or guess or request in your wildest dreams! He does it not by pushing us around but by working within us; his Spirit deeply and gently within us."

We have a relationship;

Psalms 23: 1 (NKJV), "The Lord is my Shepherd;...."

He supplies all you need; lacking nothing

Psalms 23:1 (NKJV), "I shall not want."

He gives you rest;

Psalms 23:2 (NKJV), "He makes me to lie down in green pastures;....."

He refreshes you;

Psalms 23:2 (NKJV), "He leads me beside still waters."

He healed you;

Psalms 23:3 (NKJV), "He restores my soul;...."

Jeremiah 30:17 (NLT), "I will give you back your health and heal your wounds," says the Lord."

He guides you;

Psalms 23:3 (NKJV), "He leads me in the paths of righteousness...."

He has purpose;

Psalms 23:3 (NKJV), "For His names sake."

You're tested;

Psalms 23:4 (NKJV), "Yea, though I walk through the valley of the shadow of death,...."

He protects you;

Psalms 23:4 (NKJV), "I will fear no evil;"

Psalms 91:11 (NLT), "For he will order his angels to protect you wherever you go."

He's faithful;

Psalms 23:4 (NKJV), "For you are with me;...."

He disciplined you;

Psalms 23:4 (NKJV), "Your rod and Your staff, they comfort me."

He gives you hope;

Psalms 23:5 (NKJV), "You prepare a table before me in the presence of my enemies;...."

He consecrated you;

Psalms 23:5 (NKJV), "You anoint my head with oil;...."

Give you abundance;

Psalms 23:5 (NKJV), "My cup runs over."

He blesses;

Psalms 23:6 (NKJV), "Surely goodness and mercy shall follow me all the days of my life;"

Sonja P. Davis

We're secured;

Psalms 23: 6 (NKJV), "And I will dwell in the house of the Lord...."

Psalms 23:6 (NKJV), "Forever." (*And that's eternity*).

He made a way out of no way;

Luke 1:37 (AMP), "For with God nothing [is or ever] shall be impossible."

Impossible is not in the Word of God;

Mark 9:23 (NLT), "Anything is possible if a person believes."

He is our refuge and strength

He is in control

Psalms 46:10 (NIV), "....Be still, and know that I am God;"

Provides what we need;

Jehovah Jireh (God the Provider)

Philippians 4:19 (NIV), "And my God will meet all your

needs according to his glorious riches in Christ Jesus."

Is God bigger than any problem you face?

Is God more powerful than any illness?

On many occasions; when sick, didn't the Lord heal you?

When we're broken and in our deepest pain, Lord you promise us beauty for our ashes. He'll take the burnt out mess that we experience in life and give us something beautiful.

When I was broke and didn't have enough money to pay my bills; Lord, you provided for me.

Has God ever open any doors for you, you couldn't open yourself?

Has God ever close any doors for you that no man can open? And turned around and opened a better door for you?

You've done wrong, and He forgave you.

He's a Judge in a courtroom!

When surrounded by trouble, didn't He keep you safe?

Sonja P. Davis

Protect you from danger seen and unseen?

Provide shelter in the midst of a storm?

He will give you for joy today and hope for tomorrow.

Was He there for you when you needed a friend?

When you were burden down with sorrow, did He comfort you, and hold you close, and wouldn't let you go?

Exalt His Name;

Psalms 138:2 (ESV), ".......You have exalted above all things, your name and your word."

Jesus name is above every other name

Philippians 2:9-11(NIV), "Therefore God exalted him to the highest place and gave him the name that is above every name, that at the name of Jesus every knee should bow, in heaven and on earth and under the earth, and every tongue acknowledge that Jesus Christ is Lord, to the glory of God the Father."

His name has power;

The Wheelchair Diva "In It to Win It"

John 14:13 (NLT), There's power in the name of Jesus.

Father God; according to my faith, I believe you can do anything; no matter the problem. I choose to honor you, and by faith believe that I'm healed. I believe by faith that I will walk again. I believe by faith that I'm blessed and highly favored. I will no longer be worried, stressed or frustrated, but concerned. Father God, I believe by faith, that you are working things out for my good, because Lord you said it in your Word. And I believe by faith; at the right time, in your set time, I will rise up and walk on my own; In the name of Jesus, Amen.

In Romans 8:28 Paul writes, "We know that in all things God works according to His purpose," and according to His own plan. The timing has to be right for Him to get full glory, and for you to get the utmost benefit.

Later, I was referred to Washington University in St. Louis to see a Neurologist that specializes in 'Myositis,' Dr. Alan Pestronk. He ran several tests on me as well. As a result, I'm to continue on the medication that I'm presently on. I'm to return to Frazier Rehab to have inpatient aggressive physical therapy. In fact, his medical opinions suggest that I'll be walking within 6 to 18months. He would like to see me again in 6 months, to see how I'm coming along. Truthfully, I believe the report of the Lord. He is in control. I totally depend and trust Him.

I was readmitted back into Frazier Rehab from 06/16/17 to 07/18/17 for approximately 1 month and 2 days of aggressive physical therapy.

The last time I walked on my own was August 2015. When I stood up to take steps; while walking with a walker, my legs were so wobbly. I was panicking, sweating and shedding tears. I walked 10 ft with a walker with both therapists surrounding me for protection; Kristin Little and Frannie Brohm. My legs didn't feel like they belonged to me. I kept feeling like I was going to fall forward. I was like a child learning how to walk again. Later, I was placed in a hornet which hangs from the ceiling. This was used to help me overcome fear and for safety. I walked from 20ft to 50ft. You see, I did walk. I'm asking the Lord for renew strength in my weakness. I stumbled when my knees buckled, but I regain myself, then they assisted me to sit down. I give glory to God.

I want to express my sincere appreciation for the services I received from Kristin and Frannie, also Debbie. Their help will stay in my heart forever.

I just wanted to thank them for the wonderful care and treatment they gave me from my first appointment and throughout each of the Physical Therapy sessions I received as a patient.

I want to thank Kristin, Frannie & Debbie for believing in me and encouraging me to do my best in trying new things in order to help me walk again. I have confidence in myself because of them. Also, for always having hope for me when I didn't have it for myself. And for telling me not to give up when I said I couldn't do it anymore. More importantly, for never giving up on me when I had a bad day. Their compassion gave me strength to make it another day. I am so blessed to have them as my Therapists.

As a result of their expertise and guidance, I have a much deeper understanding of Polymyositis. This rare muscle disease is what I've been diagnosed with. I have learned a great deal from them, and their involvement in my care, has helped me in becoming a Patient Advocate.

At this point, I knew it was going to be a long road ahead of me. My mind was at the Finish Line, but my body needed to catch up. I wanted to be healed and walking suddenly. I know God is able and nothing is too hard for Him. But, I must go at the pace of the Lord, and not ahead of Him; pulling Him along. I must step back and allow Him to order my steps. He knows where I've been, and He knows where I'm going. Nothing insignificant happens in your life. God uses all of it; the good, the bad and the ugly. He uses all of it for His glory.

According to 2 Corinthians 12:9 (AMP), at all times depend on God. His strength and his power work best in our weakness. He has to help us at all times to help us in all things.

Presently, I'm having Physical Therapy at one of the Frazier Rehab outpatient facilities. I'll be attending therapy twice a week for 8 weeks with Christy White. Christy is knowledgeable, credible and compassionate. She is very humble, and she communicates with me in manner that I understand. The patience she shows me reflects the type of person she is. Above all, being so supportive and compassionate aids in the success of my care. I am so grateful to have her as my Therapist.

In the interim, I'll be seeing Dr. Brown and Dr. Wagers to follow up on my progress, and to check my labs from time to time.

On September 14, 2017, I will be traveling back to St. Louis, Mo., to obtain specialized medical care and treatment from Dr. Alan Pestronk. Truthfully; it's my follow-up appointment, since I have a rare muscle disease that he specializes in. Anyway, this is my best and only option.

While waiting for that door to open, I will rejoice and continue to thank God for what He's already done in my life, and for what He's going to do in the future for me. I believe by faith he will; without question, come through for me. I don't mind waiting, for my soul has been anchored with the Lord.

**Psalms 40:1-3 (NLT) states, "I waited patiently for the Lord to help me, and he turned to me and heard my cry. He lifted me out of the pit of despair, out of the mud and the mire. He set my feet on solid ground and steadied me as I walked along. He has given me a new song to sing, a hymn of praise to our God. Many will see what he has done and be amazed. They will put their trust in the Lord."

Stay focused; Keep the Faith, and Keep Going

Conclusion

My situation may seem impossible; but God, with you, all things are possible. I got the victory when I opened up my mouth and declared by faith His promises; which is the Word of God. Watch and see how God works that difficult situation out just for me and for you too. And that's because he loves and cares for us.

You must have a relationship with God. Put God first and honor Him. By honoring Him, look out for His Goodness and Faithfulness. You get divine direction through prayer. He will lavish you with great abundance of blessings. Doors of opportunities will open up to you. You will have skills and talents you didn't know you had.

Keep running towards God. Chase after Him. Seek His face. Stay close to Him. Let favor and His light shine down on you. People will notice the hand of God operating in your life. They will want what you have. For that reason, give Him glory. Honor and praise Him, because He's worthy.

So whatever you're going through, believe you already got

the victory; believe that you've already won. Believe that good things are coming your way, and they will. Indeed, walk on with God until your change comes.

Be a credible witness for the Lord. Never forget what He has done for you. Give your testimony. Let others know how He blessed you, and how He can do the same for them.

That's what this Diva did in a wheelchair.

Somewhere over the rainbow way up high; a place where peaceful waters flow and streets pave with gold; a place where you find rest for a sin sick soul; a place I want to go. Don't you? But in order for us to get there and rest at the feet of Jesus, we must believe, we got to be saved and have a relationship with Him while down here on earth.

Pray. Believe. Keep the Faith. Stay focused. Don't keep looking back at your past, just learn from it. Stay in your lane and keep going; walking with Jesus.

Finally, when I was placing my pain to paper; on numerous occasions, I listened to Gladys. Thank you, girlfriend!

I'll leave you with these song lyrics from my favorite Artist,

The Wheelchair Diva "In It to Win It"

Gladys Knight.

"The Need to Be" - By Gladys Knight

To for-fill the need to be who I am in this world is all I ask. I can't pretend to be something I'm not, and I won't wear a mask.

There's a need to be true to myself and make my own mistakes. And not to lean too hard on someone else no matter what it takes.

I'm not fool enough to ever think that I could be the master of my fate. But it's up to me to choose my roads in life; Rocky may well be the ones I take. The ones I take.

There's the need to be something more than just a reflection of a man. I can't survive in someone's shadow; I need my very own spot to stand.

So if you're sure it's love, just be sure it's love for this thing called me. I am what I am, and I have the need to be.

In closing, stand in your truth, know that you are different and embrace it. Don't be afraid of who you are or what you

Sonja P. Davis

are.

Receive the goodness of God,

Peace,

The Wheelchair Diva

References

The Holy Bible, New King James Version, Copyright @ 1982 Thomas Nelson

The Holy Bible, New Living Translation copyright 1996, 2004, 2007 by Tyndale House Foundation

Amplified Bible, Copyright @ the Lockman Foundation 1999-2015

The Message, Copyright @ 1993, 1994, 1995, 2000, 2001, 2002

Contemporary English Version @ 1995 American Bible Society

NIV, Copyright @ 2011 by Biblica, Inc.

ESV, Copyright @ 2001 by Crossway

ERV, Copyright @ 1978, 1987, 2012 Bible League International

Good News Bible, Copyright @ 1992 British & Foreign Bible Society

Sonja P. Davis

U of L Physicians of Neurology; Dr. Martin Brown

U of L Physicians Physical Medicine and Rehabilitation; Dr. Sarah Wagers

Frazier Rehab Institute

Washington University in St. Louis School of Medicine; Director Alan Pestronk, M.D.

The Potter's House; Bishop T.D. Jakes

Oprah Winfrey-Own Network; Super Soul Sunday

Mayo Angelou

Denzel Washington

Steve Harvey

Gladys Knight

Ellen DeGeneres

Muhammad Ali

The Myositis Association; TMA www.myosits.org retrieved on August 17, 2017

Made in the USA
Monee, IL
03 December 2021

83799745R00056